SMOOTHIE FOR COLITIS

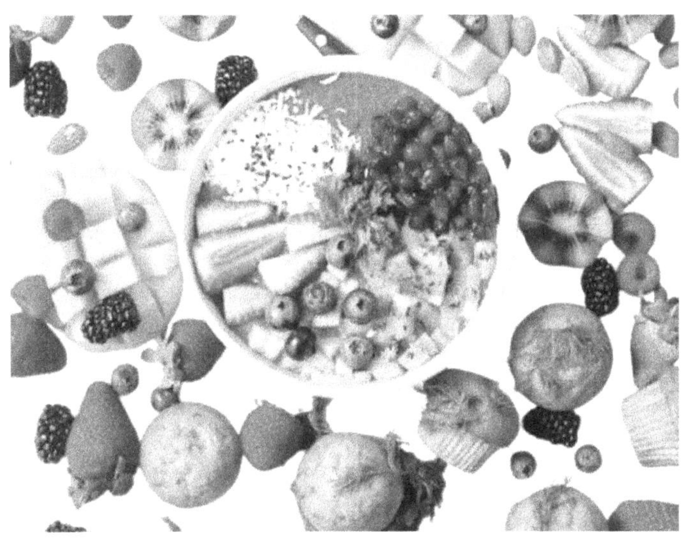

SUSAN SMITH

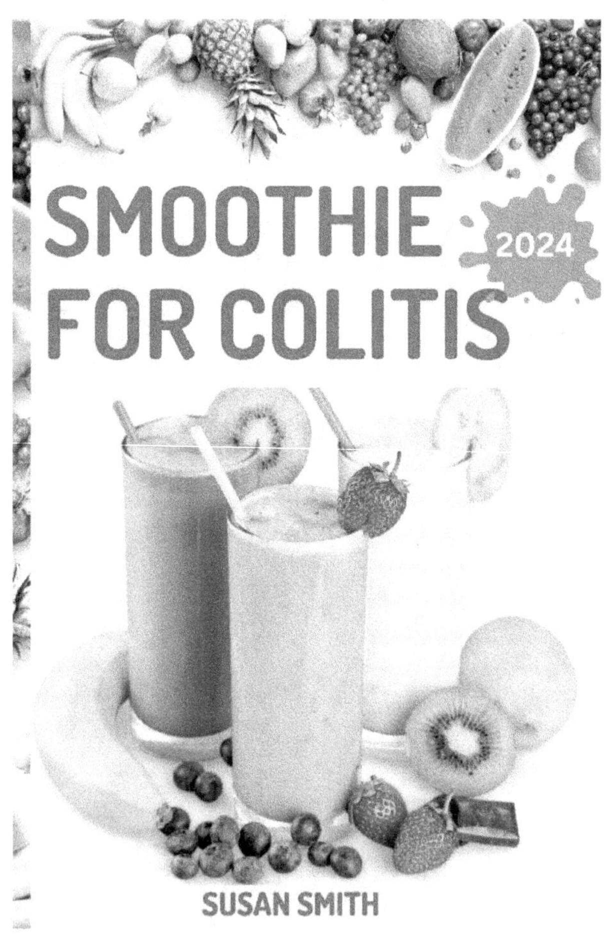
SMOOTHIE
2024
FOR COLITIS
SUSAN SMITH

TABLE OF CONTENT

INTRODUCTION

Colitis is a term used to describe inflammation of the colon, a vital component of the digestive system. This condition can manifest in various forms, including ulcerative colitis and Crohn's disease, collectively referred to as inflammatory bowel diseases (IBD).

Characterized by chronic inflammation, colitis poses significant challenges to those affected, impacting their overall well-being and quality of life.

Understanding the intricacies of colitis is essential for both patients and caregivers. The symptoms of colitis can range from mild discomfort to severe complications, such as abdominal pain, diarrhea, fatigue, and weight loss. Managing this condition requires a comprehensive approach, and one crucial aspect is nutrition.

Diet plays a pivotal role in the management of colitis, influencing symptom severity and the overall course of the disease. Individuals with colitis often experience sensitivities to certain foods, necessitating a tailored approach to their dietary choices.

 As a result, exploring food options that are easily digestible, nutrient-dense, and gentle on the inflamed digestive tract becomes imperative. This introduction sets the stage for a deeper exploration into the relationship between colitis and nutrition. By gaining insights into the nature of colitis, its impact on digestive health, and the role of nutrition in its management, individuals can make informed decisions about their dietary choices.

The subsequent chapters will delve into the benefits of incorporating smoothies into the diet of colitis patients, providing practical guidance on creating delicious and nutritionally balanced smoothies that align with the unique needs of those navigating the challenges of colitis.

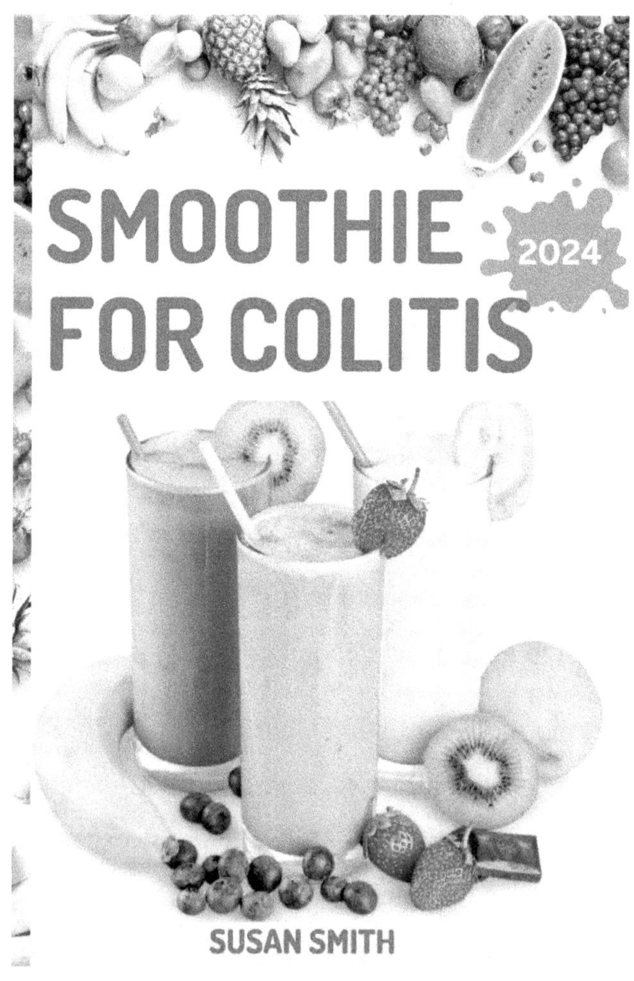

CHAPTER ONE

Definition of Colitis

Colitis, a term laden with significance in the realm of gastrointestinal health, refers to the inflammation of the colon. At its core, colitis is a complex condition characterized by the irritation and swelling of the large intestine, a vital component of the digestive system.

This inflammation can lead to a range of symptoms, including abdominal pain, cramping, diarrhea, and, in severe cases, systemic complications.

The causes of colitis are multifaceted, encompassing autoimmune factors, infections, and, at times, an elusive combination of genetic predispositions.

Understanding colitis requires a nuanced exploration of its various forms, each with its distinct characteristics and implications for the affected individuals.

Types of Colitis

Colitis manifests in diverse forms, with each variant presenting unique challenges and nuances. Among the most prevalent types are ulcerative colitis and Crohn's disease, both falling under the umbrella of inflammatory bowel diseases (IBD).

Ulcerative colitis predominantly affects the colon and rectum, leading to inflammation and the formation of ulcers on the intestinal lining.

In contrast, Crohn's disease can impact any part of the digestive tract, from the mouth to the anus, causing inflammation in a patchy and sporadic manner.

Microscopic colitis, a less common but equally impactful form, involves microscopic inflammation of the colon lining, visible only under a microscope. Ischemic colitis, on the other hand, results from reduced blood flow to the colon, posing a risk to individuals with vascular conditions.

Beyond these primary classifications, infectious colitis stems from infections caused by bacteria, viruses, or parasites. Collagenous colitis and lymphocytic colitis, both characterized by specific microscopic changes in the colon lining, round out the spectrum of colitis types.

Navigating the landscape of colitis demands a comprehensive understanding of these diverse types, each demanding tailored approaches to diagnosis, treatment, and long-term management.

By unraveling the intricacies of colitis and its varied manifestations, healthcare professionals and individuals alike can embark on a more informed and targeted journey toward wellness.

Symptoms and Impact on Digestive Health

Colitis, with its roots in inflammation of the colon, manifests a spectrum of symptoms that extend far beyond mere digestive discomfort.

At the forefront of this complex condition are abdominal pain, cramping, and persistent diarrhea, symptoms that significantly impact the daily lives of those grappling with colitis.

However, the intricacies of colitis symptoms delve deeper, painting a multifaceted portrait that encompasses not only the physical realm but also the emotional and mental dimensions of an individual's well-being.

The hallmark symptom of colitis, abdominal pain, arises from the inflammation and ulceration of the colon lining. This pain can range from mild discomfort to severe, debilitating cramps, intensifying during flare-ups and diminishing during periods of remission.

Persistent diarrhea, another common manifestation, results from the rapid transit of stool through the inflamed colon, accompanied by urgency and an increased frequency of bowel movements.

The impact of colitis on digestive health transcends the confines of physical symptoms. Fatigue, weight loss, and nutritional deficiencies often accompany the condition, driven by the body's struggle to absorb essential nutrients due to compromised intestinal function.

The perpetual cycle of inflammation and healing exerts a toll on energy levels, leading to persistent fatigue that further challenges the resilience of those navigating colitis. Yet, perhaps one of the most profound aspects of colitis is its influence on mental and emotional well-being.

The unpredictability of flare-ups, the chronic nature of the condition, and the adjustments necessitated in daily life can give rise to anxiety, stress, and even depression.

The emotional impact of colitis weaves into the fabric of an individual's identity, influencing relationships, self-esteem, and the perception of one's own body.

Understanding the symptoms of colitis goes beyond recognizing physical manifestations; it entails acknowledging the holistic toll this condition takes on an individual.

By comprehending the intricate interplay between symptoms and their far-reaching impact, healthcare professionals and support networks can foster a more empathetic and comprehensive approach to managing colitis, aiming not just for alleviation of physical distress but also for the restoration of emotional and mental well-being.

The Role of Nutrition in Managing Colitis

In the intricate tapestry of managing colitis, the role of nutrition emerges as a cornerstone, wielding profound influence over the course of the condition.

The delicate interplay between diet and colitis extends beyond the realms of sustenance, becoming a therapeutic tool that can shape the severity of symptoms, influence disease progression, and contribute to the overall well-being of individuals navigating the challenges of inflammatory bowel diseases.

Importance of Diet in Colitis Management

The significance of diet in the management of colitis lies in its ability to either exacerbate or mitigate symptoms. While dietary triggers vary among individuals, certain commonalities exist.

Foods high in fiber, particularly insoluble fiber, may aggravate symptoms during flare-ups, prompting a need for tailored dietary adjustments. Additionally, a nuanced understanding of how different nutrients interact with the inflamed colon allows individuals to craft a diet that supports healing and minimizes digestive distress.

Foods to Avoid for Colitis Patients

Identifying foods to avoid becomes a crucial aspect of colitis management. Trigger foods can intensify inflammation and contribute to symptoms such as abdominal pain and diarrhea.

These may include spicy foods, certain raw vegetables, high-fat items, and dairy products for those with lactose intolerance. By pinpointing and eliminating these triggers, individuals can exert a degree of control over the impact of diet on their colitis, fostering a sense of empowerment in managing their condition.

Importance of Diet in Colitis Management

In the intricate landscape of colitis management, the importance of diet stands as a guiding force, steering individuals toward a pathway of relief, resilience, and improved quality of life. T

he profound impact of dietary choices on colitis underscores the therapeutic potential of nutrition, transcending the mere act of sustenance to become a strategic tool in mitigating symptoms and fostering overall well-being.

One of the pivotal aspects of managing colitis through diet lies in recognizing the dynamic relationship between food and inflammation.

Certain foods have the potential to either exacerbate or ameliorate inflammation within the colon, directly influencing the severity of symptoms. By understanding these nuances, individuals can tailor their diets to create an environment that supports healing, minimizes inflammation, and contributes to long-term remission.

The customization of diets for colitis management is not a one-size-fits-all endeavor. Each individual's response to different foods can vary, making it imperative for a personalized approach.

By keeping a food journal and monitoring how specific items impact symptoms, individuals gain insights into their unique dietary triggers.

This self-awareness empowers them to make informed choices, avoiding foods that may incite flare-ups while embracing those that contribute to digestive harmony.

Fiber, a dietary component celebrated for its digestive benefits, requires special attention in the context of colitis management.

While soluble fiber can be soothing to the digestive tract, insoluble fiber may pose challenges during flare-ups. Striking a balance and tailoring fiber intake to individual tolerances become essential elements in the dietary arsenal against colitis.

Moreover, the role of diet in colitis management extends beyond the immediate alleviation of symptoms. A well-balanced and nutrient-dense diet plays a crucial role in supporting overall health, bolstering the immune system, and replenishing vital nutrients lost during periods of inflammation.

Adequate hydration, an often overlooked yet integral aspect of diet, aids in maintaining optimal digestive function and mitigating dehydration resulting from diarrhea.

The importance of diet in colitis management becomes a cornerstone in the quest for wellness. It is not merely about restrictions but about cultivating a positive and healing relationship with food. By viewing diet as a therapeutic compass, individuals navigating the complexities of colitis can forge a path toward sustained relief, resilience, and a nourished body that stands as a fortress against the challenges of inflammatory bowel diseases.

Foods to Avoid for Colitis Patients

For individuals grappling with colitis, dietary considerations become paramount in managing symptoms and fostering a sense of control over their condition. Recognizing specific foods that may act as triggers and exacerbate inflammation becomes a crucial aspect of navigating the intricate terrain of colitis management.

While individual responses may vary, certain common culprits are often identified as potential irritants, guiding individuals toward a dietary roadmap that seeks to minimize discomfort and promote digestive harmony.

1. High-Fiber Foods:

While fiber is generally celebrated for its digestive benefits, individuals with colitis may find that certain high-fiber foods, particularly those rich in insoluble fiber, can be challenging during flare-ups.

Raw fruits and vegetables, whole grains, and nuts, although nutritious, may contribute to increased bowel movements and abdominal discomfort.

2. Spicy Foods:

The bold flavors of spicy foods can be a double-edged sword for individuals with colitis.

The capsaicin in spicy foods has the potential to irritate the digestive tract, triggering inflammation and intensifying symptoms such as abdominal pain and diarrhea. Avoiding excessively spicy dishes can be a prudent step in mitigating discomfort.

3. Dairy Products:

Lactose intolerance is a common concern for those with colitis. Dairy products, rich in lactose, can exacerbate symptoms such as bloating, cramping, and diarrhea. Identifying and eliminating dairy from the diet or opting for lactose-free alternatives can be pivotal in managing digestive distress.

4. High-Fat Foods:

Foods high in saturated fats, such as fried items and certain processed foods, may pose challenges for individuals with colitis. High-fat content can contribute to inflammation and lead to difficulties in digestion, prompting a need to moderate the intake of such items.

5. Caffeine and Alcohol:

Both caffeine and alcohol can be irritants to the gastrointestinal tract. Coffee and caffeinated beverages may stimulate bowel movements, while alcohol can contribute to inflammation.

Limiting or avoiding these substances may help in maintaining digestive comfort for individuals with colitis.

Recognizing and heeding these dietary considerations empowers individuals to take an active role in managing their colitis.

While these foods may pose challenges during flare-ups, it is essential to note that individual responses vary, and maintaining a food journal can assist in identifying personalized triggers.

By navigating the landscape of foods to avoid, individuals can embark on a journey towards a diet that aligns with their unique needs, fostering a sense of control and contributing to the pursuit of relief from the challenges of colitis.

Nutritional Requirements for Colitis Patients

Colitis, with its propensity to disrupt digestive harmony, underscores the critical role of nutritional requirements in promoting healing and overall well-being.

The unique challenges posed by inflammatory bowel diseases necessitate a nuanced approach to nutrition, one that not only addresses the symptoms of colitis but also supports the body in its quest for resilience and restoration.

1. Adequate Protein Intake:

Protein, the building block of tissues and a vital component in immune function, plays a pivotal role in the nutritional requirements for individuals with colitis.

Ensuring an adequate intake of high-quality protein from sources such as lean meats, fish, poultry, eggs, and plant-based options like legumes and tofu becomes essential. Protein supports tissue repair, helps maintain muscle mass, and contributes to overall immune health, aspects crucial in the context of colitis.

2. Essential Vitamins and Minerals:

Colitis can impact the absorption of essential vitamins and minerals, leading to potential deficiencies. A focus on a well-balanced diet rich in vitamins and minerals, including vitamin D, calcium, iron, and B-vitamins, becomes imperative.

While certain individuals may require supplementation, obtaining nutrients from a diverse array of foods ensures a holistic approach to nutritional support.

3. Hydration:

The significance of hydration cannot be overstated for individuals with colitis, especially during periods of diarrhea. Fluid loss can lead to dehydration and electrolyte imbalances, exacerbating symptoms and compromising overall well-being.

Maintaining adequate hydration through water, herbal teas, and electrolyte-rich beverages becomes a fundamental aspect of nutritional care.

4. Easily Digestible Foods:

Given the potential sensitivity of the digestive tract in individuals with colitis, emphasizing easily digestible foods becomes a strategic approach. Cooked fruits and vegetables, well-cooked grains, and tender proteins are easier on the digestive system, reducing the likelihood of exacerbating symptoms.

5. Balanced Fat Intake:

While high-fat foods may pose challenges, incorporating balanced fat sources, such as avocados, olive oil, and fatty fish, can contribute to the nutritional requirements of individuals with colitis. Omega-3 fatty acids, in particular, have anti-inflammatory properties, potentially aiding in the management of colitis symptoms.

Navigating the nutritional landscape for colitis requires a personalized and informed approach. Consulting with healthcare professionals, including registered dietitians, can help tailor nutritional strategies to individual needs, ensuring a diet that not only addresses the symptoms of colitis but also supports the body's innate capacity for healing and resilience.

As nutritional requirements become a cornerstone in colitis management, individuals can forge a path toward digestive wellness and an empowered, nourished body.

Benefits of Smoothies for Colitis

Smoothies emerge as a refreshing and versatile elixir in the arsenal of dietary choices for individuals navigating the complexities of colitis.

These blended concoctions, pulsating with nutrient density and easy digestibility, offer a spectrum of benefits that extend beyond mere refreshment. In the realm of colitis management, smoothies become more than a culinary delight; they become a strategic ally in promoting digestive wellness and supporting the body's journey towards balance.

1. Easy Digestibility:

Colitis often ushers in a heightened sensitivity of the digestive system. The smooth, liquid consistency of smoothies provides a gentle and easily digestible form of nourishment, reducing the strain on the gastrointestinal tract. This attribute is particularly advantageous during flare-ups when the digestive system may be more susceptible to irritation.

2. Nutrient Density:

The core of smoothie benefits lies in their nutrient-packed composition. By blending a variety of fruits, vegetables, and other healthful ingredients, smoothies become a concentrated source of essential vitamins, minerals, and antioxidants.

This nutrient density is crucial for individuals with colitis, as it supports overall health, aids in tissue repair, and addresses potential nutrient deficiencies associated with the condition.

3. Hydration and Electrolyte Balance:

Colitis, often accompanied by symptoms such as diarrhea, can lead to fluid loss and electrolyte imbalances. Smoothies, when crafted with hydrating components like water-rich fruits and vegetables, contribute to maintaining optimal hydration levels.

Additionally, the inclusion of ingredients like coconut water or electrolyte-rich foods supports the restoration of essential electrolyte balance, promoting overall well-being.

4. Customizable and Tailored Nutrition:

The versatility of smoothies allows for a personalized approach to nutrition. Tailoring ingredients to suit individual preferences and tolerances empowers individuals to create blends that align with their unique dietary needs.

Whether incorporating protein for muscle support or focusing on specific vitamins for immune health, smoothies offer a canvas for customizable and targeted nutritional support.

5. Palatability During Flare-ups:

During colitis flare-ups, when dietary restrictions may be more pronounced, the palatability of smoothies becomes a welcome feature.

Their appealing taste and easy consumption make them an enticing option for individuals who may find solid foods challenging during periods of heightened gastrointestinal sensitivity.

In the intricate dance of managing colitis, smoothies emerge as not just a beverage but a therapeutic concoction—a sip towards digestive harmony.

As individuals explore the benefits of incorporating smoothies into their dietary repertoire, they discover a flavorful and nourishing ally that contributes to overall well-being and provides a respite for digestive systems navigating the ebbs and flows of colitis.

CHAPTER TWO

Healthy Smoothies and Juicing Recipes for Colitis

1. Berry Bliss Smoothie

Ingredients:

☐ 1 cup mixed berries (blueberries, strawberries, raspberries)

☐ 1 banana, peeled

☐ 1/2 cup Greek yogurt

☐ 1 tablespoon chia seeds

☐ 1 cup almond milk

Instructions:

☐ Blend berries, banana, Greek yogurt, and almond milk until smooth.

☐ Add chia seeds and blend briefly.

☐ Serve immediately.

Preparation Time: 5 minutes

2. Tropical Turmeric Delight

Ingredients:

☐ 1 cup pineapple chunks

☐ 1/2 mango, peeled and diced

☐ 1 teaspoon turmeric powder

☐ 1 tablespoon honey

☐ 1 cup coconut water

Instructions:

☐ Blend pineapple, mango, turmeric powder, honey, and coconut water until smooth.

☐ Adjust sweetness with more honey if needed.

☐ Enjoy!

Preparation Time: 7 minutes

3. Cucumber Mint Refresher

Ingredients:

☐ 1 cucumber, peeled and sliced

☐ 1/2 cup fresh mint leaves

☐ 1/2 lime, juiced

☐ 1 tablespoon honey

☐ 1 cup water

Instructions:

☐ Blend cucumber, mint leaves, lime juice, honey, and water until well combined.

☐ Strain for a smoother texture if desired.

☐ Serve over ice.

Preparation Time: 6 minutes

4. Spinach and Pineapple Green Smoothie

Ingredients:

☐ 2 cups fresh spinach

☐ 1 cup pineapple chunks

☐ 1/2 avocado

☐ 1 tablespoon flaxseeds

☐ 1 cup coconut water

Instructions:

☐ Blend spinach, pineapple, avocado, flaxseeds, and coconut water until smooth.

☐ Pour into a glass and enjoy the green goodness.

Preparation Time: 8 minutes

5. Blueberry Banana Oatmeal Smoothie

Ingredients:

☐ 1/2 cup blueberries

☐ 1 banana, peeled

☐ 1/4 cup rolled oats

☐ 1 tablespoon almond butter

☐ 1 cup almond milk

Instructions:

☐ Blend blueberries, banana, rolled oats, almond butter, and almond milk until creamy.

☐ Top with a few blueberries for garnish if desired.

☐ Serve immediately.

Preparation Time: 6 minutes

6. Carrot Ginger Citrus Smoothie

Ingredients:

☐ 1 cup carrots, chopped

☐ 1 orange, peeled and segmented

☐ 1/2-inch fresh ginger, peeled

☐ 1 tablespoon honey

☐ 1 cup water or coconut water

Instructions:

☐ Blend carrots, orange segments, ginger, honey, and water until well combined.

☐ Strain if a smoother consistency is preferred.

☐ Enjoy the refreshing taste.

Preparation Time: 7 minutes

7. Papaya Banana Smoothie Bowl

Ingredients:

☐ 1 cup ripe papaya, diced

☐ 1 banana, peeled

☐ 1/2 cup plain yogurt

☐ 2 tablespoons granola

☐ 1 tablespoon honey

Instructions:

☐ Blend papaya, banana, and yogurt until smooth.

☐ Pour into a bowl and top with granola.

☐ Drizzle honey over the top and enjoy with a spoon.

Preparation Time: 5 minutes

8. Almond Butter and Banana Protein Smoothie

Ingredients:

☐ 2 bananas, peeled

☐ 2 tablespoons almond butter

☐ 1 scoop protein powder (plant-based)

☐ 1 cup almond milk

☐ Ice cubes (optional)

Instructions:

☐ Blend bananas, almond butter, protein powder, and almond milk until smooth.

☐ Add ice cubes if a colder consistency is desired.

☐ Pour into a glass and savor the protein-packed goodness.

Preparation Time: 6 minutes

9. Kale and Pineapple Digestive Boost

Ingredients:

☐ 1 cup kale, stems removed

☐ 1 cup pineapple chunks

☐ 1/2 cucumber, peeled and sliced

☐ 1 tablespoon fresh lemon juice

☐ 1 cup coconut water

Instructions:

☐ Blend kale, pineapple, cucumber, lemon juice, and coconut water until well combined.

☐ Adjust sweetness with additional pineapple if desired.

☐ Serve over ice.

Preparation Time: 7 minutes

10. Minty Avocado Lime Smoothie

Ingredients:

☐ 1/2 avocado

☐ 1/2 cup fresh mint leaves

☐ 1 lime, juiced

☐ 1 tablespoon agave syrup

☐ 1 cup water

Instructions:

☐ Blend avocado, mint leaves, lime juice, agave syrup, and water until smooth.

☐ Garnish with a mint sprig for an extra touch.

☐ Enjoy the creamy and refreshing blend.

Preparation Time: 6 minutes

11. Raspberry Chia Seed Delight

Ingredients:

☐ 1 cup raspberries

☐ 1/2 cup plain yogurt

☐ 1 tablespoon chia seeds

☐ 1 tablespoon honey

☐ 1 cup almond milk

Instructions:

☐ Blend raspberries, yogurt, chia seeds, honey, and almond milk until creamy.

☐ Allow the chia seeds to swell by letting the smoothie sit for a few minutes before serving.

☐ Stir and enjoy the delightful texture.

Preparation Time: 6 minutes

12. Banana Coconut Water Smoothie

Ingredients:

☐ 2 bananas, peeled

☐ 1/2 cup coconut water

☐ 1/2 cup pineapple chunks

☐ 1 tablespoon coconut flakes

☐ Ice cubes (optional)

Instructions:

☐ Blend bananas, coconut water, pineapple chunks, and coconut flakes until smooth.

☐ Add ice cubes if a colder consistency is preferred.

☐ Pour into a glass and garnish with additional coconut flakes.

Preparation Time: 5 minutes

13. Peach Ginger Turmeric Smoothie

Ingredients:

☐ 1 cup sliced peaches (fresh or frozen)

☐ 1/2 inch fresh ginger, peeled

☐ 1/2 teaspoon turmeric powder

☐ 1 tablespoon honey

☐ 1 cup water or almond milk

Instructions:

☐ Blend peaches, ginger, turmeric powder, honey, and water or almond milk until smooth.

☐ Adjust sweetness with additional honey if needed.

☐ Enjoy the vibrant flavors.

Preparation Time: 7 minutes

14. Watermelon Mint Hydrator

Ingredients:

☐ 2 cups fresh watermelon, cubed

☐ 1/4 cup fresh mint leaves

☐ 1 tablespoon lime juice

☐ 1 cup coconut water

☐ Ice cubes (optional)

Instructions:

☐ Blend watermelon, mint leaves, lime juice, coconut water, and ice cubes until well combined.

☐ Strain if desired for a smoother texture.

☐ Serve chilled and stay refreshed.

Preparation Time: 6 minutes

15. Oat and Banana Breakfast Smoothie

Ingredients:

☐ 1/2 cup rolled oats

☐ 2 bananas, peeled

☐ 1 tablespoon almond butter

☐ 1 tablespoon honey

☐ 1 cup almond milk

Instructions:

☐ Blend rolled oats, bananas, almond butter, honey, and almond milk until creamy.

☐ Pour into a glass and garnish with a sprinkle of oats.

☐ Enjoy a nutritious and filling breakfast smoothie.

Preparation Time: 8 minutes

16. Cherry Almond Protein Smoothie

Ingredients:

☐ 1 cup cherries, pitted

☐ 2 tablespoons almond butter

☐ 1 scoop protein powder (plant-based)

☐ 1 tablespoon honey

☐ 1 cup coconut water

Instructions:

☐ Blend cherries, almond butter, protein powder, honey, and coconut water until smooth.

☐ Adjust sweetness with additional honey if needed.

☐ Pour into a glass and enjoy the protein boost.

Preparation Time: 7 minutes

17. Mango Basil Digestive Elixir

Ingredients:

☐ 1 cup mango chunks

☐ 1/4 cup fresh basil leaves

☐ 1/2 lime, juiced

☐ 1 tablespoon chia seeds

☐ 1 cup water

Instructions:

☐ Blend mango, basil, lime juice, chia seeds, and water until well combined.

☐ Let it sit for a few minutes to allow chia seeds to expand.

☐ Stir and savor the refreshing taste.

Preparation Time: 6 minutes

18. Pineapple Coconut Mint Cooler

Ingredients:

☐ 1 cup pineapple chunks

☐ 1/2 cup coconut milk

☐ 1/4 cup fresh mint leaves

☐ 1 tablespoon agave syrup

☐ Ice cubes (optional)

Instructions:

☐ Blend pineapple, coconut milk, mint leaves, agave syrup, and ice cubes until smooth.

☐ Garnish with a mint sprig for a decorative touch.

☐ Enjoy the tropical coolness.

Preparation Time: 5 minutes

19. Blackberry Avocado Smoothie Bowl

Ingredients:

☐ 1 cup blackberries

☐ 1/2 avocado

☐ 1/4 cup rolled oats

☐ 1 tablespoon honey

☐ 1 cup almond milk

Instructions:

☐ Blend blackberries, avocado, rolled oats, honey, and almond milk until creamy.

☐ Pour into a bowl and top with additional blackberries and oats.

☐ Enjoy this nutritious and filling smoothie bowl.

Preparation Time: 8 minutes

20. Lemon Blueberry Antioxidant Blast

Ingredients:

☐ 1 cup blueberries

☐ 1/2 lemon, peeled and segmented

☐ 1 tablespoon flaxseeds

☐ 1 tablespoon honey

☐ 1 cup water or coconut water

Instructions:

☐ Blend blueberries, lemon segments, flaxseeds, honey, and water or coconut water until well combined.

☐ Strain if a smoother consistency is preferred.

☐ Sip and savor the antioxidant-rich goodness.

Preparation Time: 7 minutes

21. Pomegranate Ginger Zinger

Ingredients:

☐ 1/2 cup pomegranate seeds

☐ 1/2 inch fresh ginger, peeled

☐ 1/2 cucumber, peeled and sliced

☐ 1 tablespoon agave syrup

☐ 1 cup water

Instructions:

☐ Blend pomegranate seeds, ginger, cucumber, agave syrup, and water until smooth.

☐ Strain if desired for a smoother texture.

☐ Enjoy the zesty and refreshing flavor.

Preparation Time: 6 minutes

22. Raspberry Avocado Collagen Smoothie

Ingredients:

☐ 1 cup raspberries

☐ 1/2 avocado

☐ 1 scoop collagen powder

☐ 1 tablespoon honey

☐ 1 cup almond milk

Instructions:

☐ Blend raspberries, avocado, collagen powder, honey, and almond milk until creamy.

☐ Adjust sweetness with additional honey if needed.

☐ Pour into a glass and nourish your body with collagen.

Preparation Time: 6 minutes

23. Kiwi Kale Detox Elixir

Ingredients:

☐ 2 kiwis, peeled and sliced

☐ 1 cup kale, stems removed

☐ 1/2 lemon, juiced

☐ 1 tablespoon chia seeds

☐ 1 cup water

Instructions:

☐ Blend kiwis, kale, lemon juice, chia seeds, and water until well combined.

☐ Let it sit for a few minutes to allow chia seeds to expand.

☐ Stir and enjoy the detoxifying elixir.

Preparation Time: 7 minutes

24. Peach Almond Oat Smoothie Bowl

Ingredients:

☐ 1 cup sliced peaches (fresh or frozen)

☐ 2 tablespoons almond butter

☐ 1/4 cup rolled oats

☐ 1 tablespoon honey

☐ 1 cup almond milk

Instructions:

☐ Blend peaches, almond butter, rolled oats, honey, and almond milk until creamy.

☐ Pour into a bowl and top with additional peaches and oats.

☐ Savor the delightful combination of flavors.

Preparation Time: 8 minutes

25. Green Tea Berry Infusion

Ingredients:

☐ 1 cup mixed berries (strawberries, blueberries)

☐ 1/2 cup brewed green tea, cooled

☐ 1/2 cup spinach leaves

☐ 1 tablespoon honey

☐ Ice cubes (optional)

Instructions:

☐ Blend mixed berries, green tea, spinach, honey, and ice cubes until well combined.

☐ Strain if desired for a smoother texture.

☐ Enjoy this antioxidant-rich green tea infusion.

Preparation Time: 6 minutes

26. Apple Cinnamon Flaxseed Smoothie

Ingredients:

☐ 1 apple, cored and sliced

☐ 1/2 teaspoon ground cinnamon

☐ 1 tablespoon flaxseeds

☐ 1 tablespoon honey

☐ 1 cup almond milk

Instructions:

☐ Blend apple, cinnamon, flaxseeds, honey, and almond milk until smooth.

☐ Adjust sweetness with additional honey if needed.

☐ Sip and enjoy the warm and comforting flavors.

Preparation Time: 6 minutes

27. Orange Carrot Turmeric Elixir

Ingredients:

☐ 2 oranges, peeled and segmented

☐ 1 cup carrots, chopped

☐ 1/2 teaspoon turmeric powder

☐ 1 tablespoon agave syrup

☐ 1 cup water or coconut water

Instructions:

☐ Blend oranges, carrots, turmeric powder, agave syrup, and water or coconut water until well combined.

☐ Strain if a smoother consistency is preferred.

☐ Savor the immune-boosting elixir.

Preparation Time: 7 minutes

28. Mango Papaya Coconut Bliss

Ingredients:

- ☐ 1 cup mango chunks

- ☐ 1 cup papaya chunks

- ☐ 1/2 cup coconut milk

- ☐ 1 tablespoon honey

- ☐ Ice cubes (optional)

Instructions:

- ☐ Blend mango, papaya, coconut milk, honey, and ice cubes until smooth.

- ☐ Garnish with additional mango or papaya chunks if desired.

- ☐ Enjoy the tropical bliss.

Preparation Time: 5 minutes

29. Cranberry Kale Citrus Smoothie

Ingredients:

- ☐ 1/2 cup cranberries (fresh or frozen)

- ☐ 1 cup kale, stems removed

- ☐ 1 orange, peeled and segmented

☐ 1 tablespoon chia seeds

☐ 1 cup water or coconut water

Instructions:

☐ Blend cranberries, kale, orange segments, chia seeds, and water or coconut water until well combined.

☐ Adjust sweetness with additional cranberries or honey if needed.

☐ Enjoy the vibrant and tangy flavors.

Preparation Time: 7 minutes

30. Blue Spirulina Banana Smoothie Bowl

Ingredients:

☐ 1/2 teaspoon blue spirulina powder

☐ 2 bananas, peeled

☐ 1/2 cup plain yogurt

☐ 2 tablespoons granola

☐ 1 tablespoon honey

Instructions:

☐ Blend blue spirulina powder, bananas, and yogurt until smooth.

☐ Pour into a bowl and top with granola and a drizzle of honey.

☐ Enjoy this colorful and nutritious smoothie bowl.

Preparation Time: 8 minutes

31. Soothing Green Elixir

Ingredients:

☐ 1 cucumber, peeled

☐ 2 cups spinach

☐ 1 green apple, cored

☐ 1/2-inch ginger, peeled

☐ 1 cup coconut water

Instructions:

☐ Wash all ingredients thoroughly.

☐ Chop cucumber, apple, and ginger into manageable pieces.

☐ In a juicer, process spinach, cucumber, apple, and ginger.

☐ Stir in coconut water.

☐ Serve over ice.

Preparation Time: 10 minutes

32. Berry Bliss Delight

Ingredients:

☐ 1 cup blueberries

☐ 1 cup strawberries, hulled

☐ 1 banana

☐ 1 cup almond milk (unsweetened)

☐ 1 tablespoon chia seeds

Instructions:

☐ Rinse berries and hull strawberries.

☐ In a blender, combine blueberries, strawberries, banana, and almond milk.

☐ Blend until smooth.

☐ Stir in chia seeds.

☐ Let it sit for 5 minutes to allow chia seeds to expand.

☐ Blend again briefly.

☐ Serve chilled.

Preparation Time: 15 minutes

33. Carrot Ginger Zing

Ingredients:

☐ 4 carrots, peeled

☐ 1 orange, peeled

☐ 1/2-inch ginger, peeled

☐ 1 tablespoon lemon juice

Instructions:

☐ Wash and peel carrots, orange, and ginger.

☐ Cut into smaller pieces.

☐ Juice carrots, orange, and ginger.

☐ Stir in lemon juice.

☐ Serve immediately.

Preparation Time: 12 minutes

34. Pineapple Mint Cooler

Ingredients:

☐ 1 cup pineapple chunks

☐ 1 cucumber, peeled

☐ 1/4 cup fresh mint leaves

☐ 1 lime, peeled

☐ 1 cup coconut water

Instructions:

☐ Wash cucumber and mint.

☐ Cut cucumber into chunks.

☐ Juice pineapple, cucumber, mint, and lime.

☐ Stir in coconut water.

☐ Serve over ice.

Preparation Time: 12 minutes

35. Papaya Passion Refresher

Ingredients:

☐ 1 cup papaya chunks

☐ 1 pear, cored

☐ 1/2 cup aloe vera juice

☐ 1 tablespoon honey

Instructions:

☐ Peel and seed papaya.

☐ Cut pear into chunks.

☐ Juice papaya and pear.

☐ Stir in aloe vera juice and honey.

☐ Mix well and serve chilled.

Preparation Time: 15 minutes

36. Cabbage Carrot Cleanser

Ingredients:

☐ 1/2 small green cabbage

☐ 3 carrots, peeled

☐ 1 apple, cored

☐ 1/2 lemon, peeled

Instructions:

☐ Wash and chop cabbage, carrots, apple, and lemon.

☐ Juice all the ingredients together.

☐ Serve immediately over ice.

Preparation Time: 12 minutes

37. Spinach Citrus Splash

Ingredients:

☐ 2 cups spinach

☐ 2 oranges, peeled

☐ 1/2 grapefruit, peeled

☐ 1 cucumber, peeled

Instructions:

☐ Wash spinach thoroughly.

☐ Peel and chop oranges, grapefruit, and cucumber.

☐ Juice all ingredients together.

☐ Serve immediately.

Preparation Time: 10 minutes

38. Turmeric Golden Glow

Ingredients:

☐ 2 carrots, peeled

☐ 1 orange, peeled

☐ 1/2 inch turmeric root, peeled

☐ 1/2 teaspoon ground turmeric

☐ 1 tablespoon honey

Instructions:

☐ Wash and peel carrots, orange, and turmeric.

☐ Juice carrots, orange, and turmeric root.

☐ Stir in ground turmeric and honey.

☐ Mix well and serve chilled.

Preparation Time: 12 minutes

39. Blueberry Banana Smoothie

Ingredients:

☐ 1 cup blueberries

☐ 1 banana

☐ 1/2 cup Greek yogurt (plain)

☐ 1 tablespoon flaxseeds (ground)

☐ 1 cup water

Instructions:

☐ Rinse blueberries.

☐ Peel banana and cut it into chunks.

☐ In a blender, combine blueberries, banana, Greek yogurt, flaxseeds, and water.

☐ Blend until smooth.

☐ Serve immediately.

Preparation Time: 10 minutes

40. Minty Melon Quencher

Ingredients:

☐ 2 cups watermelon chunks

☐ 1/2 cucumber, peeled

☐ 1/4 cup fresh mint leaves

☐ 1 lime, peeled

Instructions:

☐ Wash and chop cucumber and mint.

☐ Juice watermelon, cucumber, mint, and lime.

☐ Serve over ice.

Preparation Time: 12 minutes

41. Kiwi Kale Kick

Ingredients:

☐ 2 kiwis, peeled

☐ 2 cups kale leaves

☐ 1 green apple, cored

☐ 1/2 lemon, peeled

Instructions:

☐ Peel and chop kiwis and lemon.

☐ Juice kiwis, kale, apple, and lemon.

☐ Serve immediately.

Preparation Time: 12 minutes

42. Orange Carrot Cooler

Ingredients:

☐ 3 oranges, peeled

☐ 4 carrots, peeled

☐ 1/2-inch ginger, peeled

Instructions:

☐ Wash and peel oranges, carrots, and ginger.

☐ Cut into smaller pieces.

☐ Juice oranges, carrots, and ginger.

☐ Serve over ice.

Preparation Time: 10 minutes

43. Peach Almond Dream

Ingredients:

☐ 2 peaches, pitted

☐ 1/2 cup almonds (soaked)

☐ 1 cup almond milk (unsweetened)

☐ 1 tablespoon honey

Instructions:

☐ Pit peaches and soak almonds.

☐ In a blender, combine peaches, soaked almonds, almond milk, and honey.

☐ Blend until smooth.

☐ Serve chilled.

Preparation Time: 15 minutes

44. Gingered Beet Booster

Ingredients:

☐ 2 beets, peeled

☐ 1 apple, cored

☐ 1/2-inch ginger, peeled

☐ 1/2 lemon, peeled

Instructions:

☐ Wash and peel beets, apple, ginger, and lemon.

☐ Cut into smaller pieces.

☐ Juice beets, apple, ginger, and lemon.

☐ Serve immediately.

Preparation Time: 12 minutes

45. Tropical Turmeric Fusion

Ingredients:

☐ 1 cup pineapple chunks

☐ 1 mango, peeled and pitted

☐ 1/2 inch turmeric root, peeled

☐ 1 cup coconut water

☐ 1 tablespoon chia seeds

Instructions:

☐ Peel and pit mango.

☐ Juice pineapple, mango, and turmeric root.

☐ Stir in coconut water and chia seeds.

☐ Let it sit for 5 minutes to allow chia seeds to expand.

☐ Blend briefly before serving.

Preparation Time: 15 minutes

46. Apple Ginger Turmeric Tonic

Ingredients:

☐ 2 apples, cored

☐ 1/2-inch ginger, peeled

☐ 1/2 inch turmeric root, peeled

☐ 1 tablespoon honey

☐ 1 cup water

Instructions:

☐ Wash and core apples.

☐ Peel and chop ginger and turmeric.

☐ Juice apples, ginger, and turmeric.

☐ Stir in honey and water.

☐ Mix well and serve over ice.

Preparation Time: 12 minutes

47. Berry Beetroot Blast

Ingredients:

☐ 1 cup mixed berries (blueberries, raspberries, strawberries)

☐ 2 beets, peeled

☐ 1/2 lemon, peeled

☐ 1 tablespoon flaxseeds (ground)

Instructions:

☐ Rinse berries.

☐ Wash and peel beets and lemon.

☐ Juice berries, beets, and lemon.

☐ Stir in ground flaxseeds.

☐ Serve immediately.

Preparation Time: 12 minutes

48. Pineapple Basil Refresher

Ingredients:

☐ 1 cup pineapple chunks

☐ 1/2 cucumber, peeled

☐ 1/4 cup fresh basil leaves

☐ 1 lime, peeled

☐ 1 cup coconut water

Instructions:

☐ Wash and chop cucumber and basil.

☐ Juice pineapple, cucumber, basil, and lime.

☐ Stir in coconut water.

☐ Serve over ice.

Preparation Time: 12 minutes

49. Cucumber Minty Greens

Ingredients:

☐ 2 cucumbers, peeled

☐ 2 cups kale leaves

☐ 1/4 cup fresh mint leaves

☐ 1/2 lemon, peeled

Instructions:

☐ Wash and peel cucumbers and lemon.

☐ Juice cucumbers, kale, mint, and lemon.

☐ Serve over ice.

Preparation Time: 10 minutes

50. Orange Carrot Ginger Delight

Ingredients:

☐ 4 oranges, peeled

☐ 5 carrots, peeled

☐ 1/2-inch ginger, peeled

Instructions:

☐ Wash and peel oranges, carrots, and ginger.

☐ Cut into smaller pieces.

☐ Juice oranges, carrots, and ginger.

☐ Serve over ice.

Preparation Time: 10 minutes

51. Spinach Pineapple Paradise

Ingredients:

☐ 2 cups spinach

☐ 1 cup pineapple chunks

☐ 1 green apple, cored

☐ 1/2 lemon, peeled

Instructions:

☐ Wash and core apple.

☐ Juice spinach, pineapple, apple, and lemon.

☐ Serve over ice.

Preparation Time: 10 minutes

52. Mango Turmeric Sunshine

Ingredients:

☐ 2 mangoes, peeled and pitted

☐ 1/2-inch turmeric root, peeled

☐ 1 cup coconut water

☐ 1 tablespoon chia seeds

Instructions:

☐ Peel and pit mangoes.

☐ Juice mangoes and turmeric root.

☐ Stir in coconut water and chia seeds.

☐ Let it sit for 5 minutes to allow chia seeds to expand.

☐ Blend briefly before serving.

Preparation Time: 15 minutes

53. Peach Basil Breeze

Ingredients:

☐ 2 peaches, pitted

☐ 1/4 cup fresh basil leaves

☐ 1 cucumber, peeled

☐ 1/2 lime, peeled

Instructions:

☐ Pit peaches and chop cucumber.

☐ Juice peaches, basil, cucumber, and lime.

☐ Serve over ice.

Preparation Time: 12 minutes

54. Watermelon Mint Cooler

Ingredients:

☐ 2 cups watermelon chunks

☐ 1/4 cup fresh mint leaves

☐ 1/2 lime, peeled

☐ 1 cup coconut water

Instructions:

☐ Wash and chop watermelon and mint.

☐ Juice watermelon, mint, and lime.

☐ Stir in coconut water.

☐ Serve over ice.

Preparation Time: 10 minutes

55. Blueberry Spinach Elixir

Ingredients:

☐ 1 cup blueberries

☐ 2 cups spinach

☐ 1 banana

☐ 1/2 cup almond milk (unsweetened)

☐ 1 tablespoon flaxseeds (ground)

Instructions:

☐ Rinse blueberries.

☐ Wash spinach thoroughly.

☐ Peel banana and cut into chunks.

☐ In a blender, combine blueberries, spinach, banana, almond milk, and ground flaxseeds.

☐ Blend until smooth.

☐ Serve immediately.

Preparation Time: 12 minutes

56. Carrot Pineapple Ginger Splash

Ingredients:

☐ 3 carrots, peeled

☐ 1 cup pineapple chunks

☐ 1/2 inch ginger, peeled

☐ 1 tablespoon honey

Instructions:

☐ Wash and peel carrots and ginger.

☐ Juice carrots, pineapple, and ginger.

☐ Stir in honey.

☐ Mix well and serve over ice.

Preparation Time: 12 minutes

57. Raspberry Avocado Dream

Ingredients:

☐ 1 cup raspberries

☐ 1 avocado, peeled and pitted

☐ 1/2 cup Greek yogurt (plain)

☐ 1 tablespoon honey

☐ 1 cup water

Instructions:

☐ Rinse raspberries.

☐ Peel and pit avocado.

☐ In a blender, combine raspberries, avocado, Greek yogurt, honey, and water.

☐ Blend until smooth.

☐ Serve chilled.

Preparation Time: 15 minutes

58. Gingered Pear Zest

Ingredients:

☐ 2 pears, cored

☐ 1/2 inch ginger, peeled

☐ 1 tablespoon lemon juice

☐ 1 cup water

Instructions:

☐ Wash and core pears.

☐ Peel and chop ginger.

☐ Juice pears and ginger.

☐ Stir in lemon juice and water.

☐ Mix well and serve over ice.

Preparation Time: 12 minutes

59. Kiwi Berry Bliss

Ingredients:

☐ 3 kiwis, peeled

☐ 1 cup mixed berries (blueberries, raspberries, strawberries)

☐ 1/2 lime, peeled

☐ **Instructions:**

☐ Peel and chop kiwis and lime.

☐ Rinse berries.

☐ Juice kiwis, berries, and lime.

☐ Serve immediately.

Preparation Time: 12 minutes

60. Mango Coconut Green Goodness

Ingredients:

☐ 2 mangos, peeled and pitted

☐ 2 cups kale leaves

☐ 1/2 cup coconut water

☐ 1 tablespoon chia seeds

Instructions:

☐ Peel and pit mangos.

☐ Wash kale thoroughly.

☐ Juice mangos and kale.

☐ Stir in coconut water and chia seeds.

☐ Let it sit for 5 minutes to allow chia seeds to expand.

☐ Blend briefly before serving.

Preparation Time: 15 minutes

CONCLUSION

Incorporating smoothies into your diet can be a delicious and convenient way to provide essential nutrients while being gentle on the digestive system, especially for individuals with colitis.

These carefully crafted smoothie recipes aim to include ingredients known for their anti-inflammatory and soothing properties, promoting overall gut health.

However, it's important to recognize that individual responses to foods can vary, and there is no one-size-fits-all approach to managing colitis. Prior to making significant changes to your diet, especially if you have a medical condition such as colitis, it's crucial to consult with a healthcare professional or a registered dietitian.

They can provide personalized guidance and ensure that the ingredients chosen align with your specific dietary needs and restrictions. By combining these nutritious and delicious smoothie options with professional advice and careful monitoring of your body's response, you can take a positive step toward supporting your digestive health and overall well-being.